GET RID OF YOUR YOUR EYEGLASSES

Boris Tichanovsky

METHOD TO RESTORE YOUR VISION

EPAM products are one of the few healing preparations on natural basis the efficiency of which has been proved by two thousand years of practice in the past and clinical studies at the present time.

www.epam.eu

.

CONTENTS

FOREWORD

In Omsk waste lands in Siberia, in the renowned city of Bachrad, there lived Boris´s great-grandfather who was visited by people coming from all parts of Russia. Boris was an exceptional child. He had the gift to make prophecies and his parents recorded his prophecies into a special book. A great number of prophecies, concerning the life of Boris and his relations, proved to be true. He was interested in paranormal human abilities, he learnt yoga. As a schoolboy, he saw a performance of a famous fakir. After the performance was over, the fakir asked whether there was anybody among the spectators able to reproduce his tricks and Boris came to the stage and had a walk over the broken glass and lay down onto the nails. Boris repeated this performance for many years and he every time asked the spectators to have a walk over the broken glass and lie down on the nails. He was interested in their mental abilities. Nobody had to teach this art to Boris. After 15 years after the memorable circus performance, Boris became the laureate of international competition of magicians and fakirs in the city of Omlat.

When Boris organized his first course focused on sports massage, he was 16 years old. This was when he discovered his talent. After Boris finalized his school studies, he began to attend a technical university. After he graduated at the university, he was offered a job at the local department of biology. During his lectures and seminars held at this department he carried out a great number of experiments concerning biological, proving the existence and effects of such a kind of field. Then Boris exchanged the work at the department for work of a healer in the Alternative Medicine Healing Centre of Avicena. It did not take long and Boris Tichanovsky became a well-known specialist in his city of Voronez (population of a million inhabitants) and made a definite decision to give up the career of a biologist. He decided to devote his life to curing ill people. In the meantime Boris continued his studies of medicine, which he accomplished with honours. He became the manager of the Alternative Medicine Healing Centre of Avicena. He successfully passed 3 grades of Reiki under the conduct of the Dutch master of Reiki Hans Trifild, who came to Russia. Boris participated in a great number of healing courses lead by best experts. He learnt to make massage with the excellent Džuna Davitašvili, extra-sensoric medicine with Lena da Reizna, manual therapy with Kirianov, methodology of medicine with Mirzakarimov Norbekov and Larisa Fotina. He studied Chinese medicine and its arts with the Chinese teacher Tanzon and Andrej Bajramov. However, Boris Tichanovsky regards Professor Roman Zolotnicky and Albert Vasiljevič Skvorcov as his main teachers.

Boris came to Prague in 1990 for the first time. He has been working for 15 years in Bohemia as well as Russia. During that time thousands of ill people became participants of his health and healing courses. EPAM preparations helped many of them to restore their health. In the meantime Boris became master of Reiki.

Boris organizes courses on which he explains the main causes of diseases. He acquaints the people with his healing methods and their results. The participants of his courses learn how to develop abilities to activate and control their internal physical processes and how to help themselves. The courses do not only help to restore health, but also the courses make the participants happier because they learn to see the world from another perspective. The courses are conducted in a simple and practical manner and are suitable also for those people who have never met with similar exercises. Boris gained recipes for Tibetan healing preparations from his teacher Professor R. Zolotnicky and A. V. Skvorcov, inventor of EPAM. **Master Boris Tichanovsky uses 300 of these products to heal his patients.**

Get Rid Of Your Eyeglasses

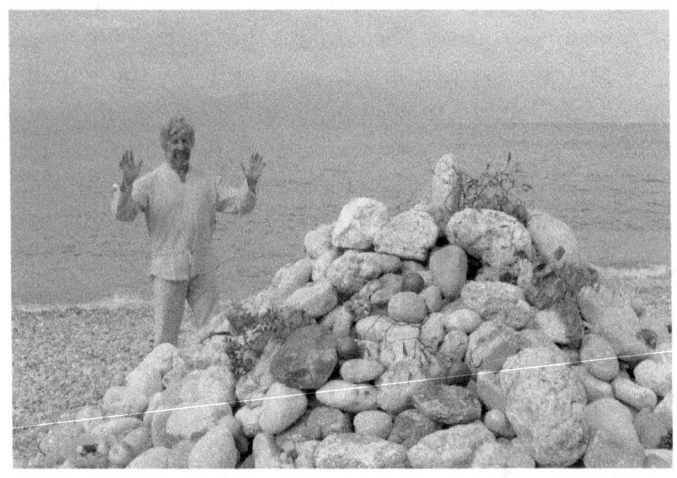

METHOD TO RESTORE YOUR VISION

I have been organizing vision restoration courses for 25 years. In 1998 I issued my first book "Help Yourself", in which I described methodology how to restore human vision to the normal. In the same year I published my other book "Secret Methods of Oriental Medicine" in Bohemia, in which the above method is mentioned as well.

This book was very brief, missing theoretical explanation. Above all, the book was determined for those who had gone through my courses for vision improvement.

Much has changed over the years however. We adapted the method for doing the eye exercises mostly in the open air, in the nature. In the recent years we have been obtaining permanent and excellent results. The vision restoration course gradually became the most popular course of all my courses in Russia as well as Bohemia (I organize many various courses: for example for regeneration of the backbone and joints, reiki, home massages, Tibetan healing methods, Thai and Chinese massages, taj-czy cjuaň courses, courses focused on digestive system and female organs, trance techniques courses and many others.).

I am absolutely sure that the theory is correct because right selection of the theory has influence on how the things are afterwards put into practice. Only practice can show whether things are correct. Many years of organizing the courses proved that the method is very efficient. After a week vision of the most participants has reached improvement of 1 – 2 dioptres. If the participants continued to do the exercises according to my recommendation even after end of the course, the process of improvement continued.

Vision improved or completely recovered even in such serious cases of eye diseases as glaucoma, cataract, retinal detachment, optic nerve diseases and others. I decided to describe this unique method of regeneration and complete recovery of vision including theoretical explanation. The reason for this was that I wanted to make this method and vision restoration available also to those people who did not attend any vision restoration course.

Many years of observation proved that the improvement is permanent. If you follow our advice your vision shall not impair in the course of time, but – on the contrary – it shall improve.

The description of the method in this book is so detailed that it can be practised not only by the participants of our courses but also by all those who want to restore their impaired vision or keep their vision in a good state.

I am very glad that also the people with good vision can acquaint themselves with this method. If man respects the following recommendations, he can preserve his vision to old age. I recommend that already school-children should learn this method because this is the only way for most people to preserve good vision for life.

The courses are attended by people with impaired vision, yet this book is intended also for those with good vision.

Let those who have the ears hear – let those who have the eyes see...

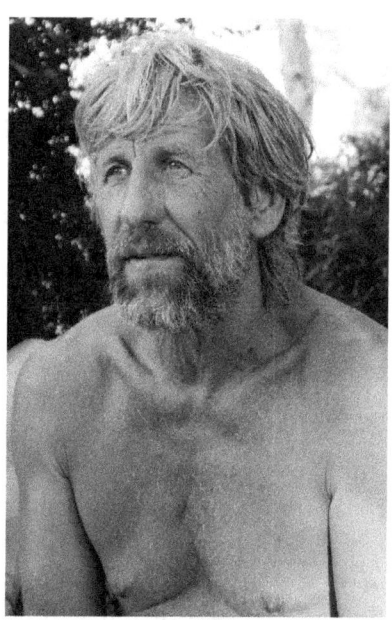

THEORY

If you have ever been dealing with vision, you must have read books by William Bates and his followers and you know his method. I will not reproduce this method because we have found a more straightforward method of vision restoration. I will mention just the most important points on which we base our method.

At the beginning of last century American ophthalmologist William Bates proved that exercises can improve and restore human vision, thereby eliminating the need to use eyeglasses. This conclusion was fundamental. His numerous followers continue his work and vision restoration centres are run according to the method by William Bates in many countries around the world.

William Bates discovered the reason why vision tends to impair. By his opinion, this tendency is mainly caused by the fact that we are trying to see better than our eyes are able to, which means that we overstrain our eyes thereby forcing them to focus. This excessive pressure causes that our eyes impair. Our emotions play an important role as well: negative emotions contribute to the tendency that our vision impairs. When William Bates endeavoured to find out a method how to improve vision by means of exercises, he discovered the mechanism of accommodation, which is the ability of the eyes to see near as well as distant objects. At the time of Helmholtz it was still believed that the process of accommodation is realized only by the lens. If the curve radius of the lens changes, the focus length changes as well, which makes the fixed object to project right to the retina. Thanks to this mechanism we can see both distant and near objects clearly. This means that the process of accommodation is influenced by the changed curve radius of the eye lens. Nevertheless William Bates proved that there exists another mechanism of accommodation: changes of focus length inside the eye can also be caused by the fact that the muscles distributed around the eye adapt the shape of the eye, thereby also changing its focus length. Large eye muscles have the ability to correct vision without using eyeglasses, by correcting malfunction of the eye lens. The large eyes muscles are easy to train. William Bates introduced a great number of exercises and procedures which can help people recover their vision. The most of the exercises were not invented by William Bates – instead he found them in hatha yoga, which dates back several thousands of years ago.

Another contribution to the theory and practice of vision recovery was delivered by Mirzakarim Norbekov and Larisa Fotina. You may have read their book "Healthy and Young For Ever" or the book by Norbekov "How to Get Rid of the Eyeglasses", "Fool's Experience or Key to See the Things Right"). M. Norbekov and L. Fotina were not focused on the emotions which causes vision impairment, but they were rather interested in the emotional states which can help us to restore our vision. Certain emotional states which can be evoked intentionally and any exercises for the eyes (and not only for them) are much more efficient. These authors came up with psychophysical exercises for vision restoration, which we are going to acquaint ourselves with. The both authors used the secret Muslim yoga as the source of information.

William Bates as well as M. Norbekov used the same source of information which has existed for several thousands of years. William Bates proved already a hundred years ago that it is possible to restore human vision by means of exercises. Groups of William Bates´ followers are active in many countries. In the recent time several methods have been devised by various authors which advise how to restore vision. Also, courses are held and books issued which describe these methods. However, there emerges a question why, in fact, more and more people wear eyeglasses and contact lenses and why eye surgery is so widely practised. There exist two main causes of this. The first one is in contradiction with the global official medical science. Since the time of Helmholz ophthalmology derives its profit from money of the companies producing eyeglasses and lenses. This includes scientific research, technical equipment, professional training and salaries paid out to physicians. Since eye surgery became a profitable business, most physicians (as they are taught at universities) ignore alternative possibilities of vision restoration. Another cause consists in the fact that the method by William Bates and other authors is rather laborious. In order to achieve good results it is necessary to make an effort and to devote much time to exercises – however man is, by nature, lazy. So it is much easier to put on eyeglasses. All known methods of vision restoration are a "long-distance run". I pay tribute to William Bates, who was a man of genius. Nevertheless, the most serious mistake of the authors which base their work on the concept introduced by William Bates is the fact that they spend most time by doing the exercises indoor. We have, however, found a shorter way how to restore human vision.

This way was shown to me by my teacher, Medicine Professor Roman Zolotnicky, who lived in Tibet for many years, where he learnt Tibetan medicine and Tibetan yoga. I myself have not devised anything as well, but my vision restoration course is conceived on the basis of Tibetan yoga and Tibetan medicine and also the well-known methods by William Bates, M. Norbekov, L. Fotina and other authors.

What is the most important about my method? Professor Roman Zolotnicky revealed some very interesting knowledge to me, which I would like to explain briefly. The scientists observed primitive tribes around the world, which lived in primitive communal society. These are isolated regions of the central Africa, regions along the Amazon River in the Latin America, some tribes living in reserves in North America, some nations living in the north of Russia and some tribes living in Australia and other regions. Since the scope of these observations is very wide, I will not describe them in detail. We are interested in the scope of problems related to human vision, which was a part of the research carried out. As expected, the people of the above nations and tribes have excellent ability of vision, which is preserved to old age. Their vision is much clearer than vision of European people. If we assign the value of 1 to the quality of the vision of an average European, the quality of vision of the above primitive people can be described by the value of 1,5 – 1,7. They do not suffer from eye diseases such as cataract, glaucoma and others, which is self-understandable: they do not write, perform calculations, do not overstrain their eyes at work, they do not watch television, and they do not work with computers. It is natural that their vision is excellent. However, our interest is focused on something else. When the scientists watched and scrutinized video materials recorded during the research, they noted a matter of interest: eyes of these people keep in permanent motion. More close observation showed that the eyes of these people fix every object for an average duration of 2 seconds. The scientist assumed that the 2 seconds is an optimal period of time within which the eyes move from one object to another. So, it is optimal for the eyes from the viewpoint of physiology.

I will leave the (from our viewpoint) primitive tribes and I will devote my attention to Buddhist monks living in Tibet. The monks spend the major part of time by reading, learning and making handwritten copies of holy books, very often by candlelight, which means by poor light. From this reason, the eyes of the monks are overstrained, maybe more than the eyes of European people. Despite this fact, most monks keep their excellent vision to very old age. How can we explain this? Every day the monks regularly do eye exercises, always in the open air, in the nature, where they can watch the horizon in the distance. When the scientists made a video recording of the Buddhist monks doing their exercises, they were surprised by the following fact: during the exercises the eyes of the monks were in permanent motion. It was ascertained that the average space of time for which the eyes of the monks stayed fixed on a single object, is two second, which means the same as in the case of the primitive tribes mentioned above. Is that a strange coincidence? - No, it is a rule. Two seconds are, from the physiological viewpoint, an optimal time during which the sight is moved from one object to another. This is why the everyday exercises are sufficient for the monks to keep their excellent vision for their life.

Let us get back to our vision restoration method. I have mentioned that my method draws ideas from the work by W. Bates, M. Norbekov, L. Fotina and some other authors, however it is mainly based on the studies carried out by Professor R. Zolotnicky, Tibetan yoga and Tibetan medicine.

Here are my conclusions:

* I tell you just like W. Bates: in order to work properly our sight needs both sunlight and absolute darkness. W. Bates introduced exercises in which the eyes are exposed to sunlight (solarisation – gaze at the sun) and exercises in which the eyes are in absolute darkness (palming). He took over these exercise from yoga. I will explain the exercises in detail later on.

* For comfort and health of our eyes we need to keep them in permanent motion during the day for a certain period of time. In order to restore impaired vision it is important for the eyes to keep in permanent motion for as long space of time as possible. Optimal time during which we move our eyes from one object to another are 2 seconds. It is necessary for the eyes to get accustomed to this rhythm.

* All eye exercises must be done in the nature, especially in the places where man has a distant outlook, best of all, where man can see the horizon. It is not by a mere chance that the Tibetan monks train their eyes only in the places where they can see the horizon.

* Our eyes benefit from natural green colour of plants: grass, foliage, needles. This is why man should direct his eyes to vegetation in the summer and to coniferous trees in the winter.

What we are doing now is not doing exercises – we are just learning to use our eyes properly.

The aim is to avoid waste of time. We are all busy and we feel a need to chat with our neighbours in the street or with our friends on the phone for several hours, to watch another part of an endless popular serial on TV and to do many other "important" things. In order to minimalize the time necessary for vision restoration, we need to develop a conditioned reflex: once we have left our home, we must learn to use our eyes properly. On weekends and holiday we should devote as much time as possible to our health and our eyes. What do we, in fact, mean under the phrase "use our eyes properly"? This means to use our eyes in the manner how the God intended us to do and how the Nature arranged for the eyes to be used. Some scientists suppose that man has been inhabiting the world for about 30 thousand years, the other suppose that for several millions of years. Compared to these spaces of time, system writing was invented relatively a short time ago. This is why it is ideal for our eyes if we are walking through an eye-pleasing nature and if we are using our eyes in a *jumping* manner, *sliding* manner, *panoramic* manner and in a combination of these.

Jumping sight – we gaze at an object for the duration of 2 seconds

Sliding sight – Our eyes are, in a steady pace, sliding from one object to another, which means that the eyes are in a permanent and smooth motion

Panoramic sight – we gaze forward, to an empty space. In order to learn to use our eyes in a wide field of vision, we need to learn to use our peripheral vision.

The ability to use our eyes properly is the most important thing that is taught in the courses. We should use our eyes properly whenever we are in the open air. It is important and sufficient for our vision to be restored. All the exercises are to be done in the state of meditation, in which the exercises are maximally efficient. The state of meditation has many rules, the most important of which is the "promise of silence". We always keep this promise during the exercises done in the courses although some participants feel this difficult. If man is talking and doing exercises at the same time, it seems to him that he is consistent. However, in reality he does nothing properly. We have another important task for you: when doing exercises, you should stop your logical mode of thinking and switch to imaginative mode of thinking, which means thinking in terms of images and ideas, not words. Our body works as follows: the brain controls all its subordinate organs according to the rule "who does not work shall not eat". This can be explained like this: if man has a broken arm or leg which is immobile in a plaster cast, after a certain time the muscles will get weak, the limb will start to accumulate salts and waste products of metabolism, which means that the limb will turn into a "pit for waste material". If the limb is immobile for too a long time, the ability of motion can be lost for ever, the limb can get "dried-up" and turn into a bone covered with skin. The brain supplies nutrition only to those organs and parts of the body that are working.

And what about human vision? The things are the same. Here is a vicious circle: if our vision impairs, the brain will start to receive less information, which causes that the brain will reduce the quantity of nutrition supplied to the eyes. We can however outwit our brain and we can force our brain to supply as much nutrition to our eyes as possible. How can we do that? I will explain. I do not like the human brain to be compared to a computer, however this is very illustrative in this case. If we take fifty thick books from the library and if we re-type them to the computer, it will take relatively little space in its memory. If we take large high-resolution colour photos or a video films (animated pictures), we will need more memory in order to save them into the computer. Man may think that the books contain much more information, however they take much less memory, whereas the pictures will take ten times as much memory. The conclusion is the following: if man wants to be erudite and if man is studying and memorizing all possible scientific books all day long, only 10 to 20 % of our brain works. The rest of the brain is idling because it gets no information. The brain says to itself: "What is going on? There is no information, there is nothing to do, which is boring". Nevertheless if we start to use our imaginative mode of thinking, it seems to us that we are doing nothing, just strolling and enjoying the nature, but our brain receives much more information, for which the brain is most grateful.

There are a great number of factors which play their part in this process, which will be discussed later on. Now it is important to understand that when strolling in the nature, enjoying this, we are able to switch over from logical mode of thinking to imaginative mode of thinking and our brain will start to receive much more information, in exchange for which it will give our eyes all what our eyes need, i.e. the brain will create ideal conditions for our eyes to work properly.

Another piece of information for you: one of the methods of improving weak memory and sclerosis is travelling. This is why tourism of old people is very widespread in developed countries. What is the benefit of travelling? Man arrives at a certain place in order to learn its history and beautiful nature. When travelling thinking spontaneously switches from logical mode to imaginative mode and the brain receives ten times as much information as normally. Thanks to this, the brain and the body begin to get younger. This fact however does not mean that we have to travel because everybody does not have financial means to do so. There is beautiful nature also in our surroundings and so it is enough to go out and enjoy the natural beauties around us. It is important not to speak and think over any plans, dismiss any problems, thereby gradually entering into the state of meditation and learning how to think in an imaginative mode. This will enhance brain activity, launch the process of rejuvenation of the brain, body and vision restoration.

Let us come over to another issue, which is the question why we cannot see. The God gave us the eyes in order to make us happy - but happy about what? About the God´s work. The God created the Earth for us with its mountains, oceans, seas, rivers and waterfalls. The God created the skies with the stars, plants and animals on land so that we, his beloved children, can rejoice in this.

We receive some 80% of information from the surrounding world by means of our eyes but we have ceased to enjoy this. Most people, people with impaired vision above all, do the following mistake: when they leave their houses, they do not enjoy the sunlight, blue skies, white birches or flowers below the window – instead they are gazing below and so they can see cigarette stubs, plastic beer bottle under the bush and so they will get angry: "What kind of a scoundrel has created such a mess here?". Then they will take a look at the road and they can see potholes in the asphalt: "What is the bloody municipal administration doing?" Then they see a rusty car in the street: "This is the last straw! What kind of an idiot did something like this? He has a car but he cannot take care of it." In this way all his life passes by, day by day. We do not see its beauty but, instead, we can see jut the ugly things. This is why our eyes do not enjoy their ability to see.

In order to restore your vision, the first thing you have to learn is to rejoice in what you can see. Rejoice when you see a yellow maple leaf, bunch of red rowanberries, white clouds in the sky because this all is God´s work. What can be more beautiful than live nature? Just compare a live flower with an artificial one. Learn to find beauty which is around you. Learn to notice what surrounds you. When walking, we have got accustomed to look just below, to see a coin two meters in front of us, but all the other things are ignored by us. I emphasize again: in order to restore our vision it is above all important to look carefully at everything around us, to learn to find beauty and rejoice in it.

Now I am going to make a few notes about eyeglasses. What are their disadvantages? Once we put them on, the field of our vision gets reduced at once. This means that the range of the eye movement will get reduced as well (tunnel vision). If the range of motion is reduced, the muscles will get shorter and blood formation will get impaired, which has a negative impact on the process of nutrition process of the eyes. To explain the things better, I will use the following example, which I usually present in my courses. Imaging you need to chop up wood but this must be done in a specific manner: sweep of the axe must not exceed half a meter. What will happen? Within half an hour you will get very tired, your hands will get sore and you will not manage to chop up the wood. If the swing of the axe is to be ten centimetres, the axe shall fall out of your hands after five minutes of work. If you chop the wood using the full swing, you will be able to work for hours, you will enjoy this, you will chop up enough wood and, in addition, you will feel joy because your muscles are working properly. The same rule also applies to your eyes: if the muscles work in the full range of motion, they relax regularly, which supports blood formation and process of nutrition. If the muscles do not work in the full range, they gradually get stiff and blood formation as well as nutrition will get impaired. Once we put on eyeglasses, the blood formation and nutrition of the eyes will get yet more impaired, which will worsen their state.

And now let us devote ourselves to contact lenses. Contact lenses very often cause allergic and inflammatory responses with all the related consequences.

We will pay attention also to another aspect of eyeglasses and lenses. Opinion of Professor of medicine, ophthalmologist Oleg Pankov has proved to be right. This physician, who devoted majority of his life to curing eye diseases, published results of his long-time practice in curing vision in the book "Murderous Eyeglasses", from which I take the following citation: "Sunlight is necessary for the eyes. The sun shall preserve the healthy eyes in a good state, and will improve impaired vision. The sun will support metabolic processes in the eyes and get the eyes rid of waste substances. Besides, our eyes and body need ultraviolet radiation. All the people wearing eyeglasses are in fact chronically ill and suffer from various diseases, not only those afflicting the eyes. This is caused by the fact that the organism of these people does not continually absorb ultraviolet radiation. Note the fact that only 20% of ultraviolet radiation is absorbed by the skin during the year whereas 80%

by the eyes. The glass of the spectacles and lenses do not let ultraviolet radiation through." This is an opinion of a scientist, professor of medicine and ophthalmologist.

This all applies to common eyeglasses. However what do people say about tinted sunglasses? First of all let me remind you of the tales presented in advertisements suggesting that man cannot live without sunglasses. Tale one: in the recent years the solar activity has increased considerably. However, the truth is that the solar activity regularly increases and decreases and our eyes have got adapted to this process in the course of millennia very well. Tale two: owing to chemical industry the ozone layer of the Earth is getting depleted, thereby creating ozone holes, which enable direct space radiation to penetrate the atmosphere. Again, this problem is not as serious as described. The ozone holes come into being over the South and North poles of the Earth, where the Earth gravitation is lower. This is why if we are to travel to these geographical regions, we should make sure to take tinted sunglasses with us. Where else can we need tinted sunglasses? In the mountains, in the altitude above three thousand meters above the sea. When skiing, we need protective glasses against wind and snow, but we do not need glasses against ultraviolet radiation.

I will leave the topic of human vision for a while and I am going to say a few general words on negative influences. Some "would-be" scholars like to scare people as follows. The sun: too intense activity, direct radiation. The Earth: impaired magnetic field. Soil: polluted by chemical waste and exhausted. Air... Water... Altogether, get yourself ready for your grave, lie down and wait for your death.

Man is protected against all these negative influences by several protective shields which surround him. The God has given us the ability to protect ourselves such as the ability to heal ourselves. Live and enjoy your life.

Let us get back to common eyeglasses and lenses. What? To put them off right now and leave them for ever? - By no means. Instead we can make our eyes gradually adapted to life without eyeglasses and lenses or we can step by step reduce the dioptre value of our eyeglasses and lenses. From now on we will put off eyeglasses and lenses whenever we can do without them. I have mentioned that the main cause of vision impairment is the fact that we force our eyes to see more clearly than they are able to see. This means that if we need to have a close look at something, for example when reading, working with PC, we can put the eyeglasses on. But when walking, we can do without the eyeglasses without any problems. In our courses of vision restoration held in the open air the people can do without eyeglasses even in the case of values ± 6 dioptres. I remind the fact that the majority of time during the course is spent in the open air. An important challenge is to learn how to do without eyeglasses whenever it is possible but, at the same time, to have the possibility to use them when it is important.

As a rule vision of the participants of the courses begins to improve already during the course itself. Most people will improve their vision by 1 – 2 dioptres within a week. If man follows the rules of our method, this improvement of vision continues even after end of the course. It is very important to change the eyeglasses and lenses at the right time so that the process of improvement should not be reverted.

Now a few words about how to check our vision. Vision checks are done by means of various tables used by ophthalmologists. Depending on the type of the table, vision is checked for the distances of 1, 3 or 6 meters. These tables were invented a very long time ago, which will be mentioned later on. If we check our vision by means of such a table, we will learn what we in fact are able to see. In the recent years ophthalmologists started to use medical devices which measure how eye lens work. Some hundred years ago, W. Bates proved existence of another mechanism of accommodation which works by means of changed shape of the eye. This mechanism can easily be trained. In fact we do not care according to what principle our eyes work and what accommodation mechanism they use. More important is what ability of vision we have. This is a story of one of the people who participated in our course: the participant noted that his vision had considerably improved – he was able to read text in the newspaper without eyeglasses, which he could not before, he was able to see very distant object, which he could not before. Therefore he visited his ophthalmologist, who measured his vision acuity by means of a technical device. The ophthalmologist told him: "The things are the same as they were before, there is no improvement. Do not trust your eyes, trust me."

We endeavour to obtain evidence from our ophthalmologists proving that our vision has improved. Such improvement was in many cases confirmed by measuring technical devices, however the improvements ascertained by such equipment were mostly smaller than they were in reality. This is why we recommend you to check your vision with the use of the tables.

Now we will deal with our vision from another aspect. I would like to share some of my conclusions which I draw during my practice of a healer in the course of many years. On consultations with my patients I very often use manual therapy and I also work with the backbone. I came to a conclusion that there are people whose vision is good but they have problems with their backbone. However there do not exist people with bad vision but healthy backbone. People with bad vision have very often problems also with their cervical spine (backbone of the neck). This is why in order to restore vision it is important to cure up the backbone first. Manual therapy, application of needles and massage will help to improve the state of the backbone very fast but the main factor in curing the backbone are, undoubtedly, special exercises. In my work I use various sets of exercises for curing the human body. I am quite sure that the best set of exercises for curing the backbone and joints is the set by M. Norbekov and L. Fotina. The exercises described in this set are also taught in our courses. Besides the courses, you can acquaint yourself with this set in the book "Secret of Life or Help Yourself", on the video cassette "Medical Treatment of the Backbone and Joints" or in the book by L. Fotina "Lora".

Apart from exercises for improving our backbone, we also need to learn how to keep our body in the right posture. What does "right posture" mean and how to learn to maintain it? I tried to find the answer in professional medical literature on health and sports. What do these "expert" books say? They contain a detailed description of the suffering which are ahead of you if your posture is not right. Also, the professional books contain definitions of right and wrong postures, one author citing another. The most frequented instructions how to keep your body properly is the following: "Stand with your back pressed to the wall, press your heels and nape to the wall too, put your arms behind your back so that the back of your left hand rests on your lower back and the back of your right hand rests on your left palm. If your right palm touches the wall, your posture is right. If there is a gap between the palm and the wall and if the hands are not in contact, your posture is wrong." This method is absolutely absurd because it is suitable only for individuals of average height, neither thick nor thin, with athletic figure. According to this method, all thin, thick, tall and small people are supposed to have wrong posture. Besides other similar methods I came across there also exist other, quite useless, instructions such as "do not arch your back, sit and stand upright" etc.

In Tibet this question was solved a very long time ago in an ingenious and simple manner (everything ingenious as also simple). The perfect posture means the position in which our body is "growing". We are to pull ourselves upwards, but at the same time we must remain quite relaxed. The process of our growing is imaginative rather than physical, done by our muscles. You should above all concentrate on the fact that you must not raise your shoulders. It is necessary to combine two aspects: to pull yourself upwards but, at the same time, remain relaxed. In this manner man must stand, sit and walk. When sitting, we do not lean our lower back or the shoulder against the edge of the desk at all. In order to keep your posture right, follow this rule: try to keep your sight at the level of your eyes.

Try to maintain the right posture right now. Stand up, pull the top of the head upwards like a flower reaching for the sunlight, keep relaxed, keep your vision at the level of your eyes, feel the freshness of your body and smile. Remember the position in what your posture is right because this position is unique just for you. Try how it feels if your posture is right when sitting and then try to maintain it also when walking.

If your posture is right, your physical energy circulates through the channels properly, your blood formation is functional and distribution of your internal organs is good as well. Maintaining the right posture also helps you to be in a good mood.

It is time to talk about curing emotions. This is really not a mistake – I really mean "curing". M. Norbekov and L. Fotina proved that in some emotional states the curing exercises and procedures are considerably more efficient than in a situation when man is in a normal emotional state and much more efficient than in the case of negative emotions. The above authors called this state "*image of youth and health*".

Image of youth and health is a little "bit" of happiness which everybody has ever experienced in his life. Here are examples of such a state:

* You have won a football match played in the courtyard, which made you happy for a while. You will forget your broken knee and the homework you have to do. At this moment you like yourself and the others like you.

* For the first time in your life you feel that you can swim.
* For the first time in your life you can see sunrise.
* At dancing courses you met a very beautiful girl (partner) and she (he) is smiling at you.

There are many of such joyful moments and it is possible that you can remember several of them. I myself keep several of this kind of moments in my mind.

* Snow and the sun. I am skiing in the mountains, together with a beautiful girl. I am flying like wind, I can feel pleasure and I am doing everything very well.
* Dancing floor. I can hear popular piece of music and I am dancing with the girl I love.

What happens with man if he is in such a state? If we imagine youth and health, i.e. if we are experiencing a "bit" of happiness, we feel extraordinary emotional enthusiasm and freshness in all our body, we like ourselves and the others like us. We dismiss pain and problems (if we have any) and the only thing we are doing at that moment is that we are enjoying our life. When we evoke this *idea of youth and health* in our mind, the exercises will get much more efficient. In order to get into this state, let us recollect our happy moments and let us live them again. Let us recall as many details of that moment and state as possible: weather, music, clothes, sweet smells and, above all, physical feelings.

When doing exercises try to evoke the *idea of youth and health* as frequently as possible. Another thing. Much has been written about the very important role of smiling. In the civilized world people learn how to smile. Smiling is healthy, but I disagree with the so-called "American" manner of smiling in a uniform style, which is a matter of fashion. Your smile should reflect the state of your mind and this is why you should learn to smile with your eyes. Nobody is able to smile with his eyes if he cannot feel his smile also in his soul. And his smiling mouth is just an addition to his "smiling" soul.

The last issue I intend to mention in the theoretical part is game. Everything we are doing in our courses is a kind of game. Everything I am telling you is just a fairy-tale. When doing exercises man should not overstrain himself but instead he should just be playing a game. When a child plays, he or she does not exert himself or herself but still he or she is doing everything all right. It is not by a mere chance that Gospel says: "be like children and you shall be blessed".

This is all the practice and theory concerning my vision restoration method. The theory has been explained in details so that you know what you are doing, why you are doing that and how you shall do that. If you know the theory, you yourself will be able to restore your vision. I want to share my fund of experience accumulated for many years during my vision restoration courses with you. The courses are attended by people with various disorders of vision. The process of vision restoration is easiest and fastest in the case of people who were born with good vision and who developed impaired vision (short-sightedness or far-sightedness) in the course of their life by abusing their eyes or because of their wrong style of living. The restoration will also be effective in the case of inborn defects of vision but it is necessary to put more effort and time into doing the exercises in order to achieve vision restoration. Vision will improve or be entirely restored in the case of the following eye diseases: glaucoma, cataract, retinal detachment, optic nerve atrophy. We do the same exercises and procedures in the case of all the above diseases. How is it possible? The reason is that in my courses I do not cure diseases of the eyes or vision disorders themselves, but instead I teach the participants how to move their eyes correctly in the manner as intended by the nature and the God. I teach my pupils to keep their eyes constantly in their physiological optimum, which brings them maximum benefit.

By means of exercises and procedures, state of meditation and the most important instrument – emotions – we are going to restore blood formation and eye nutrition process to the normal state, which will cure up our eyes and restore our vision in all the case of vision impairment.

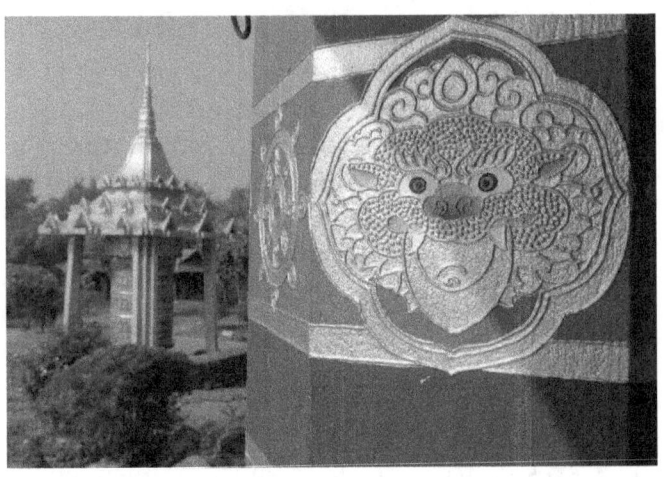

PRACTICE

Our main exercise is *jumping look*. I remind that the look will move from one object to another in a period of 2 seconds, which is ideal for the eyes from physiological point of view. The exercise is done when sitting, standing or walking. Types of *jumping look*.

1. Palm - distance

Stand up. Hold the arm bent in the elbow so that the flat palm is stretched out at a distance of some 50 cm in front of your eyes. We gaze at the palm for 2 seconds, then we take a look at any distant object which we can see or we simply look at the horizon. Again, we watch our palm for 2 seconds and then we gaze into the distance for 2 seconds. We do this exercise for 3 – 7 minutes. Doing it, we select a different distant object each time. During the 2 seconds we collect some information about this object: its colour, shape etc.

Another variation of this exercise: we cover one of our eyes with the palm in the same manner as when doing palming (palming will be mentioned later on). The other eye observes the palm for 2 seconds. Then we look into the distance for 2 seconds. We do the exercise for 2 – 3 minutes. Then we exchange the eyes.

2. Below at our feet - distance

We are looking at the ground, at the distance of a step in front of us, for 2 seconds, then we look into the distance for 2 seconds. Each time we choose a different object both on the ground and in the distance, on which we focus our eyes. The exercise is to be done for 3 – 7 minutes.

Another variation: we do the exercise with one eye for 2 – 3 minutes, then with the other eye again for 2 – 3 minutes. We cover the idling eye with the palm.

On principle, the exercise is to be done when walking.

3. Below, at the feet – To the left, distance – Below, at the feet – To the right, distance – Below, at the feet – To the front, distance

The exercise is to be done the same way as the previous one. We look below, at the feet for 2 seconds, then we turn the eyes maximally to the left and look into the distance for 2 seconds, then 2 seconds below, at the feet again. Then we turn our eyes maximally to the right and look into the distance for 2 seconds, and again for 2 seconds below, at the feet and in the end we will look forward for 2 seconds (e.g. at the horizon). The exercise is to be done for 5 – 15 minutes. We do this exercise even if we are moving or walking.

Another variation: when doing this exercise, we cover either the right or the left eye.

General rule: If the right and the left eye have different defects, we should devote more time to train that eye which is impaired more seriously.

4. To the left, distance – To the right, distance – Upwards, distance

We will keep the eyes in the same vertical level as they are and we will turn the eyes to the left, to the right, upwards, but we will never look downwards. We move the eyes every 2 seconds. We do the exercise for 5 – 15 minutes. We do the exercise when moving or walking.

All these exercise are variations of jumping look and can be freely alternated.

Before I teach a new exercise to you, I am going to tell you a fairy-tale.

Once upon a time, very long ago, there governed the king called "Hrach", who loved warfare best of all the things. He waged endless wars and this is why he needed more and more soldiers. Men were recruited to the army and so they started to think over how to dodge this military service. For example when a certain man was asked to join the army, he said: "My vision is bad, I cannot distinguish our soldier from a soldier of our enemy and so I could shoot one of our soldiers." Therefore the King's advisors invented the same tables for vision examination as the physicians are using at the present. But the tables did not help. They asked the recruit: "Can you read it?" and showed him the smallest letter in the lower part of the table. "No, I cannot read it". So they showed him the biggest letter in the upper part of the table. "I can see something." How to force the recruits to tell the truth? The King got angry and told his advisors: "If you do not think out something more practicable, you yourself will be recruited to the war." Then personal physician of the King came up with the following trick: "Follow my thumb," said to one of the recruits and slowly and fluently raised his thumb upwards and then downwards, to the left and then to the right. He himself observed the recruit´s eyes. When the eyes were moving smoothly and regularly, it meant that the recruit´s vision is excellent so the recruit was forced to join the army. If the eyes were moving in a jerky, spasmodic manner, it meant that the recruit´s vision was in fact bad. The jerkier the movement of the eyes was, the worse the vision was. Quivering pupils indicated a nervous disease. Such a soldier would not be good.

This method has been used up to now by the physicians. The only change is that nowadays a small bar is used instead of the thumb. You must have met with this method of vision examination yourself.

Why are the eye movements smooth if vision is good, whereas why are the movements if vision is impaired? The eyes are able to move smoothly and without spasm only if the ocular muscles are relaxed. If they are strained, in cramps, the eyes move in a jerky, "jumping" manner. The cause and the consequence are the same. If we learn to move our eyes smoothly, our vision will be restored to the normal state. If we try to move our eyes smoothly, we learn to relax them at the same time.

Let us learn this. We will start with *jumping look.*

5. Jumping look to the left – to the right

We turn our eyes maximally to the left and then smoothly, without interruption, to the right. Then we return back, which means to the left. We turn the eyes to the right for 8 seconds, and then to the left for 8 seconds. The eyes do not stop in the out positions. The most important is to keep the eyes constantly directed into the distance. We repeat the exercise for 3 – 7 minutes without break. Ask somebody to tell you how your eyes are moving. This exercise can also be done in a fast pace and with one eye covered. We do this exercise also when moving or walking.

6. Sliding the eyes upwards – downwards

We look at the ground and then we are moving the eyes upwards, to the sky, smoothly, slowly and without interruption, for a period of some 8 seconds. Then, without interruption, we move the eyes downwards for about 8 seconds, to the ground. This exercise can also be done in a fast pace or with one eye covered. The exercise is done for 3 -7 minutes. We do this exercise also when moving or walking.

7. Sliding the eyes along a fan-shaped path, forwards and backwards

Look at the ground, about a meter in front of your feet, and then direct the eyes into the distance for a period of 4 seconds. Doing it, note all the objects which get into your field of vision. Then return your eyes back to your feet for a period of 4 seconds and note all the objects which get into your field of vision. Look into the distance but to a different point and then return the eyes to your feet again. In this manner, look into the distance in a different direction (always start from the same point). We do this exercise for 5 – 15 minutes. We do this exercise also when moving or walking.

8. Sliding the eyes along a spiral path

Look into the distance at any object and then move your eyes in a sliding matter along a spiral to the left, then for 1 second perceive as large field of vision as possible. When doing it, note everything around you. Then return the eyes along a spiral path to the most distant object and note all the objects on the path. Then change the direction of the eye movement to the right and repeat the exercise. We do this exercise for 3 – 7 minutes. We do this exercise also when moving or walking.

All these exercises are variations of *sliding look*. You are free to alternate between two or more exercises of *sliding look* and between an exercise of *sliding look* and an exercise of *jumping look.*

Exercises for restoration of proper function of the vestibular system.

If we put on eyeglasses, our field of vision gets narrower and functioning of the vestibular system gets is impaired. This is why much attention in our courses is devoted to training vestibular system.

9. Turning the head to the left – to the right

We are walking forwards and keep turning the head maximally to the left and to the right. The most important about this exercise is to look into the distance and observe the most distant objects. Doing it, you can use *jumping* or *sliding look.* As a variation, you can also do this exercise when walking backwards. Do the exercise for 1 –5 minutes.

10. Making circles with the head

We are walking forwards and making circles with our head smoothly. Doing it, we are looking into the distance and observing our surroundings. We can use *jumping* or *sliding look.* As a variation, you can also do the exercise when walking backwards. Do the exercise for 1 –5 minutes.

11. Turning backwards

We are walking forwards and turning our body backwards to the left shoulder and then to the right shoulder. We are looking backwards into the distance for 2 – 3 seconds. We do the exercise for 1 –5 minutes.

12. The chin up and down

We are walking and tilt the head maximally backwards and then forwards so that the chin touches the chest. When looking to the ground, we note flowers and grass, when looking to the sky, we note clouds.

13. Turning

We slowly and smoothly turn the body to the left 4 times and then to the right 4 times. Doing it, we are looking into the distance and looking out for eye-catching objects and also everything around us. The exercise can also be done when walking. We do this exercise for 3 – 7 minutes.

Exercise for improving peripheral vision

Peripheral vision can save our life. We are in deep thought, gazing without concentration, crossing the street and suddenly we catch sight of a car which emerged from the curve. You say that you know this situation? Eastern fighting arts devote much attention to developing peripheral vision, which enables man to see all the surrounding space at once.

14. Looking at the fingers

We join the thumbs of the right and left hands. We raise the joint thumbs to the eye level, at the distance of 20 – 25 cm in front of the eyes, then we touch the tip of the nose and then we remove the joint thumbs to the original distance of 20 – 25 cm. At the end we touch the point between the eyebrows. We do the movement smoothly and our eyes follow the thumbs. Then we separate the thumbs and move them aside towards the ears, looking forwards with our peripheral vision perceiving the both thumbs (we are trying to put the thumbs maximally to the sides). We move the fingers in order to control them better. The exercise is to be repeated 3-4 times.

15. Peripheral vision

We walk along a path in the forest, looking into the distance and observing the trees along the both sides of the path. Our peripheral vision is not clear, but instead we can see just contours. We do this exercise for 10 – 15 minutes.

16. Panoramic sight

We look into the distance where we can see open space. Then we close the eyes and then we image and draw what we saw. We close and open our eyes repeatedly.

17. Watching the world with the eyes open wide

As mentioned, people wearing eyeglasses have got accustomed to narrow their eyes. Have a look at the people around you in order to see that this is true. We need to get rid of this bad habit. When narrowing the eyes, we are watching the world through narrow slits, which makes the field of our vision yet narrower. If we keep our eyes opened wide, our field of vision becomes wider. Imagine you are watching TV. Now open your eyes wide and imagine the cinema screen. Can you see that difference? Start walking with the eyes opened wide. Keep your field of vision as wide as possible.

We have just reached a very important exercise.

18. Combination of the panoramic and the sliding look upwards – downwards, along a fan-shaped path

Panoramic look means that the field of vision has the maximum possible width, the eyes being opened wide. Keeping the visual field as wide as possible, we glide with our eyes forwards and backwards along a fan-shaped path.

Let me brush up how to do the movement along fan-shaped path. We move the eyes from our feet into the distance for about 4 seconds, then we move the eyes back to our feet for about 4 seconds. The eyes are moved smoothly, noting the near as well as distant objects. Then we repeat the same gliding movements, but in the opposite direction, keeping our visual field as wide as possible, i.e. we are combining wide-field look with jumping look upwards – downwards along a fan-shaped path.

Participants of our courses paint landscapes with aquarelle technique. We need not master this technique (I myself am not a good painter but I like painting pictures). I ask the participants to make a painting of what they saw. At the end of the courses their paintings are much better than those created at the beginning of the courses. Many a time the paintings at the end of the courses are very good.

Our lessons combine exercises using jumping, gliding and panoramic look. When doing the exercises, we learn to breath, wink the eyes frequently because this helps the eyes to be relaxed. To reach relaxation we also use the technique of palming.

PALMING

Palming is a gift for your eyes. It is an ideal exercise to relax the ocular muscles and the eyes. Do it every time when your eyes are tired. The more frequently, the better.

It is done as follows: rub your palms against one another until they get warm. Then put the palms to your eyes so that no light gets through to the eyes. First, keep the eyes opened in order to make sure that you can see absolute darkness, then close the eyes and imagine the darkness.

When doing palming, keep your eyes closed. Relax the strain in your fingers, relax the wrists and elbows. Lean against the knees or the table so that your nape and backbone are in a straight line. You can put a pillow under your elbows on your knees. If you need to be bent forwards, bend yourself in the waist but keep the nape and the backbone in a straight line. The manner in which the palms are put to the eyes will be individual. Find the position which is the most comfortable for you.

This exercise is important above all because it make the eyes relaxed. The ocular muscles get relaxed, which activates their nerve cells. This relaxes the strained muscles which turn the eyeballs and keep the eyes in the axis. Also, it gives energy to the optic nerve and the retina nerve. If you do palming after you exposed the eyes to sunlight, you keep them closed until the retina nerves absorb the sunlight. Do palming for about the same duration as you did the solarisation (see later on). This will provide the eyes with power and health, which in most cases will restore your vision.

19. Palming – phantasy

When doing palming, imagine something beautiful what you saw or what you would like to see. I will give examples.

* Imagine the see, waves with white foam. You are looking into the distance and you can see a boat with red sails, which you find amazing. The boat is leaving until it disappears beyond the horizon. You are enjoying the beauty of the cliffs, partly covered with woods.

* Now we are skiing in a snow covered forest. The green branches of spruces and pines are bent down under the snow load. Snow and the sun, fresh air.

* Now we are in a summer forest. On a clearing, there are very many tiny suns – blooming dandelions. We will pick up a bloom. There is an ant creeping along the stem. We are scrutinizing the ant, we are looking at its small legs, antennas, eyes. Our vision has never been so good and clear. We carefully blow the ant down to the grass and smile with happiness.

20. Palming – listening to the birds

When doing palming in the nature, the best practise is to listen to birds singing. If the birds are not singing, we can listen to other natural sounds: babbling brook sounds, rustling foliage etc.

21. Palming – music

When doing palming, try to enjoy ear-pleasing music.

The vision centre of the human brain is connected with the hearing centre and this is why if the hearing centre is activated by pleasing sounds also the centre of vision is activated.

22. Palming – warmth of the hands

Before doing palming, rub consistently the palms until they get warm. When doing palming, concentrate yourself on the warmth and imagine the warmth flowing from the palms through the eyes to the brain.

After doing palming, you will find the surrounding world clearer and nicer.

Do palming several times a day whenever your eyes need relaxation. Do palming after every single solarisation.

SOLARISATION

William Bates describes solarisation as follows. The eyes need absolute darkness just as well intense light. If you want to cure and keep your vision, practice solarisation whenever it is possible.

The technique of solarisation is simple. Above all, it is important to put off the eyeglasses and contact lenses. Stand at the margin of a dark shadow, either in the corner in your home or in an illuminated doorway. Put one of your feet on the dark (not illuminated) spot on the land and the other foot to a spot illuminated by intense sunlight. Close your eyes and take a deep breath, start to turn the head from side to side so that your closed eyes pass through the space in the shade and the space which is flooded by intense sunlight. Hold your head in such a manner that the sunlight goes straight to the point between the eyelids of the closed eyes and the eyebrows. When turning the head, keep saying to yourself: "The sun is coming, the sun is leaving." Keep turning the head until the eyes start to shiver and hurt.

Expose your face to intense sunlight, keeping the eyes closed. Now, start turning your head and the body, in a relaxed manner and without strain, to the right, to the left, raise your heels off the ground, saying to yourself: "The sun is passing to the left and to the right around me, to the left and to the right again, every time in the contrary direction than I turn my head." It is very important about what you are thinking when doing solarisation because it can hinder the movement of the eyes under the eyebrows of the closed eyes and also it can make difficult for you to look at the sun during the exercises. Let the sun go around you.

Once the eyelids cease to shiver, once the eyes cease to be narrow when directed to the sunlight, and after the eyes begin to feel comfortably when making the turns, cover one eye with the palm so that absolutely no sunray can get through. Put the palm to the eye in such a manner that the covered eye may be open. Now start turning the head, slide the look of the uncovered eye along the ground in front of your feet. Doing this, keep winking the eye. Now, raise the head and the elbow, turn from side to side, winking the eye quickly, gazing directly into the sun. You will be surprised by the fact that this exercise, despite sensitivity of your eyes, does not hurt you and by the fact that you can tolerate the sunlight very well. Repeat the exercise with the other eye. In the end do the exercise with both the eyes simultaneously. Turn the head and direct your closed eyes right to the sun. Here the solarisation ends. You will see flickering in front of your eyes, colour spots and suchlike, caused by the sunlight. Therefore go to shade and do palming for twice as long time as you did solarisation.

Once your eyes start to accept the sunlight

without problems, you will be flooded with pleasant feeling of physical comfort. The feeling of freshness and psychic relaxation will stay. Dark room will not give you half the feelings which you can get thanks to sunlight.

From the viewpoint of physiology hardening the eyes is priceless because the eyes will cease to suffer from reflections of the sun on the surface of lakes, very bright snow or dazzling reflection of the sun in desert sand. Also, your eyes will start to feel comfortably, e.g. when dazzled by car headlights if you live in the city. For the eyes to feel comfortably, it is very useful to relax the retina nerves, which will enable us to tolerate light of any intensity.

Keep also in mind that the sun enhances the visual capability of the retina nerves and the eye nerve, which will help you to understand that the sun is a "somebody" to make friends with. Once we understand that the sun keeps the eyes healthy, improves the metabolism of our vision and the eyes, eliminating waste products from the eyes, we can appreciate the benefit of sunlight. The physicians are always surprised to see the light rose-coloured, healthy and solarised retina which is different from the normal, pale eyes, suffering from the lack of sunlight. From the viewpoint of aesthetics, the sun makes the eyes lively and shining, in which the sun cannot be substituted.

Do not do solarisation when wearing eyeglasses or lenses otherwise you will injure your vision. During the course, we practice solarisation several times a day. Otherwise it is sufficient to do it once a day, in the summer and winter. Now I am going to describe how we practice solarisation in our courses.

23. Universal solarisation

This type of solarisation can be done whenever during the year and in any part of the day: at noon, in the morning or evening, on a day without clouds as well as on a day when the sky is clouded.

Expose the face to the sun, cover one eye with the palm like when doing palming, do not touch the eye, and keep the other (opened) eye winking. Turn the whole body smoothly from side to side. Raise your look from the ground upwards, into the sun. Fix your look at the sun and turn the body a few times, keep the winking eye directed to the sun. Then start to lower the look to the ground. Raise the look and then lower it to the ground several times. We do solarisation for 2 – 5 minutes. When the sun is too intense and if your eyes are over sensitive to light, stop the movement of the eyes before reaching the sun (below the sun) where you do not feel unpleasant feelings.

24. Solarisation at sunrise and sunset

Depending on individual visual feelings, you can look into the sun with both the eyes without winking or turning the body, about 40 minutes - 1 hour after the sunrise and the same time before the sunset. You will find the time of sunrise and sunset at the calendar because in the mountainous the sun can appear above the horizon later and disappear below the horizon earlier.

25. Solarisation at weak sun

If the sun is partly covered by clouds, we will start to do universal solarisation. Afterwards we look into the sun with both the eyes, we wink the eyes and turn the body. If the sun is hidden behind the clouds, we need not wink the eyes but still it is necessary to turn the body and do solarisation like at sunrise.

The eyes will always suggest which type of solarisation you are to do. During solarisation, you must not have unpleasant, painful feeling in the eyes.

26. Sky solarisation

If the sun is covered by thick clouds and if you can see clean blue sky between the clouds, we can practise universal solarisation. Doing it, we look at the parts of the clean blue sky, not into the sun.

27. Passive solarisation

When the sunlight is intense, we can practise solarisation with the eyes closed. We are looking into the sun with the eyes closed and, doing it, we can turn the body. The maximum duration of solarisation is 5 to 20 minutes. This type of solarisation can be done also when sitting. After solarisation, perform some kind of palming. You should do palming for leastways the same time as you did solarisation. Your eyes will suggest how long the palming should be. If you cover the eyes with the palms after solarisation, you will see spots of various colours in front of your eyes. Keep doing palming until the colour spots which you can see settle down.

LARGE TURNS

William Bates described this exercise as follows. Approach a window in the room, keep your feet at the width of your shoulders. Shift the weight of your body to the left leg, turn the head and shoulders to the wall on the left. Then shift the weight of the body to the right leg and turn the head and shoulders to the wall on the right. Do the exercise in the pace of a slow waltz and, in each turn, raise the respective heel off the ground. If you are singing a melody of a pleasant waltz, you will find out that you are breathing deeply. Note that the windows are flickering as you are turning your look. Do not let this motion to hypnotize you – just imagine the relationship between the movements: you and the windows are passing by. Let the windows pass by you. If you fix your look to the windows, you head will be spinning and you will get sick.

When your look passes by the windows, make sure to keep your eyes opened, otherwise you will not see the windows passing by you. Count the number of the turns. In order to reach the necessary degree of relaxation, make 60 turns. Between the turn 60 – 100 enjoy the relaxation, in which your vision starts to improve.

This exercise is to be done 100 times in the morning and 10 times in the evening before going to bed. Despite the fact that it does not take more than 2 – 3 minutes, you will be surprised by its effects. This exercise makes the backbone mobile and normalizes functioning of the internal organs (heart, lungs, digestive tract etc.). Above all, it evokes unique vibrations in the eyes (very tiny, spontaneous movements of the eyes) with the frequency of about 70 movements per a second. You yourself understand that vibration of such frequency cannot be induced intentionally. This can be proved just by the seeming movement of the windows when making the turns.

Keep in mind that this exercise is not intended to be a physical training but it is to strengthen your vision. Its aim is to relax the eyes and make them move in accordance with your thoughts. Besides, this exercise is to remove the bad habit to fix objects with the eyes for a long time. Do the exercise in a relaxed, rhythmic manner, do not make it as a physical training. The turns are to bring about relaxation and rid the body of strain. Keep this in mind.

We modified the exercise in the courses as follows.

28. Large turns

Spread your feet at the width of your shoulders, keep the feet parallel. Turn the body in a relaxed pace to the right and to the left with maximal range of motion. Keep the feet to the ground. The most important is to be absolutely relaxed. Look into the distance but try not focus on anything. Let the surrounding objects pass by your eyes. Do the exercise with the eyes opened for 1 – 3 minutes. Then do 4 turns with the eyes opened and 4 turn with the eyes closed. Do the exercise for 2 – 5 minutes. Then close the eyes and devote yourself to the movement. Do the turns with the eyes closed for 5 – 10 minutes. Like all the other exercises, also the large turns are to be done in beautiful nature with a distant outlook.

29. Making turns in front of the index finger

This exercise is another step to eliminate the strained eyes. Place one of your index fingers in front of your nose. Turn the head from side to side slowly, but do not look at the finger. It will seem to you that the finger is moving. Soon the floor may start to move under you and so close your eyes and turn so that the tip of the nose touches the finger every time when passing by. If you look at the finger after you open your eyes, you will feel dizzy and you lose your balance.

Can you not see any illusion of motion? If you really cannot see anything like this, do the following. Put your palms to your face, spread your fingers wide. Turn the head and imagine that the fingers are a kind of small bars which the head is passing by. Do not look directly at them, but through them into the distance. Do 3 turns with the eyes closed and 3 turns with the eyes opened and observe the fingers passing by you. Keep saying to yourself: "The bars are moving to one ear, to the other ear…" Do 20 – 30 turns and keep breathing in mind.

This exercise eliminates pain. If you have headaches or any other aching, do the turns for 10 – 20 minutes and alternate them (with the eyes opened and closed). Then do palming and you will feel a relief. Keep thinking on the motion which is happening in front of your eyes.

30. Winking the eyes when breathing in

We wink the eyes three times every time when breathing in. When breathing in, we have the eyes closed. We wink and close the eyes in a relaxed manner, without strain. We do this exercise for 1 – 3 minutes.

31. Narrowing the eyes when breathing out

We narrow the eyes every time when we breathe out. When breathing out, we open the eyes wide. We do this exercise with a light strain. This exercise is to be done for 1 – 3 minutes.

32. Meditation breathing

It is our common manner of breathing by the nose. We breathe in a colder air, which gets warm in our body and is breathed out warm. This temperature difference is several degrees in the summer and several tens of degrees in the winter. Anybody can easily feel the difference of 1 – 3 degrees. Realize that if somebody has fever of 39 °C and if you put your hand on this forehead, you will say: „He is heating as a stove." This is why we need to concentrate ourselves just on the temperature difference between the air which is breathed in and the air breathed out. Now it is the most important thing of all. When breathing in, we can feel cold within our nose, when breathing out we can feel warmth. When breathing in we can feel cold and freshness within the nose, when breathing out we can feel warmth and pricking. Slow down breathing a little bit in order to feel the difference between the warmth and cold better. Now imagine that you are breathing with your eyes. The body does not exist, there are only beautiful living eyes, which are breathing. When breathing in we can feel cold and freshness within our eyes, when breathing out we can feel warmth and light pricking. Breathing with the eyes is very pleasurable.

The meditation breathing is to be done for 2 – 10 minutes.

33. Psychophysical exercises for the eyes

When the ocular muscles are strained, the nutrition of the ocular muscles and all the ocular tissues is impaired.

In order to restore vision it is important to restore blood formation and nutrition of all the ocular tissues to the normal. We use special psychophysical exercises, based on the idea of warmth, cold and pricking in the respective spots.

When the feeling of warmth is evoked the blood vessels get wider, which increases the blood flow rate. When feeling cold, the blood vessels get narrower and the blood flow rate gets lower. In this manner blood formation and tissue nutrition in the given places can be enhanced considerably as proved by studies carried out using medical apparatuses. When we evoke feeling of pricking, nerve endings get activated.

Imagine sunlight on your nape, caressing the nape with its rays. When breathing in, draw warmth, pricking and burden from the nape. Conduct this warmth to your eyes and warm your eyes with every time when you are breathing out. Send the warmth back to the nape. Now your nape is fanned by cooling breeze. When breathing in, draw cold and freshness from your nape and send the cold and freshness to your eyes. Wash your eyes with this cold and freshness, with this living water. After you did this exercise, check your vision by means of medical tables and you will certainly mark improvement.

MEDITATION

The technique of meditation is described in detail in our books „Secret Methods of Oriental Medicine", „Secret of Life" and meditation calendars for the third millennium.

W. Bates noted that under the given circumstances vision tends to get impaired, above all, in the case of the people who are responsible, ready to accommodate other people, putting much emphasis to fulfilling tasks and in the case of people with unstable psyche and in the case of pessimists.

Restoration of vision needs positive emotions. This is why meditation is a very important part of our courses. We have worked out unique methods of meditation. For the purpose of these meditations, Jelena Tomilinova created special esoteric pictures. We recorded a few audio and video cassettes with our meditation. A Moscow publishing house issued an album of meditation pictures "Enlightenment", which is of premium quality. In Bohemia a meditation calendar with pictures by Jelena Tomilinova was issued. You can use the calendar and audio cassettes for your meditations.

Get Rid Of Your Eyeglasses

PROCEDURES

As I have mentioned several times, our main task is to relax the ocular muscles, restore blood formation and nutrition of the eyes. Besides the exercises which we learnt we will use other simple procedures that will help us. The procedures are alternating washing of the eyes with cold and warm water, clay warm and cold masks, warm and cold compresses.

Alternating washing of the eyes

In restoring blood formation and eye nutrition, the following contrasting water procedures are helpful.

34. Alternating washing of the eyes – variation 1

This variation is simpler and most frequently used in the courses. We turn the cold-water tap on. We sprinkle the cold water on our face with the eyes closed for 10 – 20 seconds. Then we open the hot-water tap, adjust the temperature to a pleasant value (37 – 42 °C) and sprinkle the warm water on the closed eyes for 10 – 20 seconds. We alternate the warm and cold water several times. The duration of the procedure is about 2 minutes.

35. Alternating washing of the eyes – variation 2

We full two washbasins with water of the temperature 18 °C and 36 °C. We wash our eyes for 1 minute, alternating between the cold and warm water. We exchange cold and warm water 5 – 7 times. We can gradually increase the temperature difference up to 10 °C and 40 °C. If your eyes are oversensitive, you can dissolve a bit of salt in the water – 1 teaspoon in 1 litre of boiled water. We can also modify the duration of washing from a few seconds to a quarter of an hour.

36. Clay masks

Clay masks are put on the eyes, the eyes being closed. The temperature of cold masks is 10 – 20 °C, the temperature of warm masks is 38 °C. After quarter of an hour, the masks are washed off. We can apply first a cold mask and then a warm mask (each for the duration of quarter of an hour). We can however use only one mask: cold or warm. Follow your intuition. You should feel comfortable with the mask on.

37. Compresses

For warm compresses, lukewarm or warm water is used. Alternatively the compresses can also be dry, in the form of a woollen scarf. We can also use an electric pillow. Cold water, ice or snow are used for cold compresses. Cold or warm compress is to be applied for the duration of 10 – 15 minutes and we alternate between them.

A general rule is: we start the day with a warm compress in the morning. We end the day with a cold compress. Before sleep we begin with a cold compress and we end with a warm compress. Also, we can apply one compress, cold or warm, for 15 minutes every day and follow our intuition.

FOOD

Common varied food is the kind of food you are accustomed to. We only recommend to eat more fruit, vegetables, walnuts (Lombard walnuts, almonds, walnuts, pine nuts etc.)

Carrot, hippophae and rosehip juice are healthy too. The food should include cheese, curds, meat and eggs.

EPAM Skvorcova 1000 will help you to restore your vision. For vision restoration use the clay mask with mumio called "Reviving".

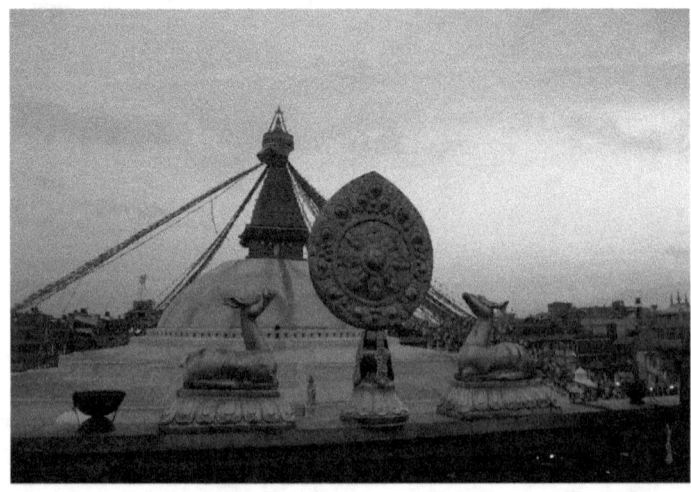

AFTERWORD

All the exercises for vision restoration are to be done in the state of meditation (promise of silence). Doing the exercise, we try to *imagine youth and health* as frequently as possible. Most important is to enjoy what we see and learn to find beauty around us. We do the exercises in beautiful nature, forest, park where we have a distant outlook and where we can see the horizon. The efficiency of the exercises is much higher if they are done in the nature than in the case that they are done indoors.

Our eyes need both sunlight (solarisation) and absolute darkness (palming).

We learn to use our vision properly, especially when we are in the open air. When we are on courses, we spent the major part of the day in the open air. People with impaired vision usually fix objects for a long time: they fix a point for 5 – 7 second and then fix another point etc. On the contrary we learn to use *jumping look, sliding look, panoramic look* and combinations of these. Doing the exercises we learn to see the world as we used to do formerly.

If I should explain the method of vision restoration in other words, I would say: we help the eyes to recall the ideal physiological state when the eyes were in permanent motion.

The first week, we need to get rid of unpleasant feelings in the eyes when doing the exercises. When doing the exercises, we feel something like sand, light dull pain and suchlike in the eyes. It is the same as in the case of muscles: If they are trained, the will start to get relaxed but painful at the same time. This is why we need to re-train our eyes to get them relaxed and to launch the mechanism of vision restoration. In order to launch the mechanism of restoration, we train the eyes for 3 – 4 hours a day in the nature the first week. After a week, unpleasant feelings in the eyes will disappear. We follow the rules of using our vision I have mentioned (*jumping look, sliding look, panoramic look* and their combinations) whenever we go out (to work, from work, to shop, for a walk) leastways once a day. Dedicate a free day to your soul and your body. On the free day take a walk in the nature, following our advice and enjoy your life for leastways 2 – 3 hours. Do not waste the free day watching TV on the couch or doing the dusting.

It is not by a mere chance that Gospel says: work for 6 days and dedicate the seventh day to the Good. Dedicate your free day to the God, soul and body.

Keep your backbone in your mind. The backbone is a system which needs your permanent attention. We recommend that you should train your backbone every day, especially in the morning, whenever you are free.

Remember the simple helpful procedures. We recommend you to do the alternating washing of the eyes twice a day, in the morning and evening. The other procedures are to be done once or twice a week.

This method is, at the present, the fastest way to restore your vision. It has been used by thousands of course participants with the aim to restore their vision. Now, also you have the same opportunity.

Go and reach your destination.

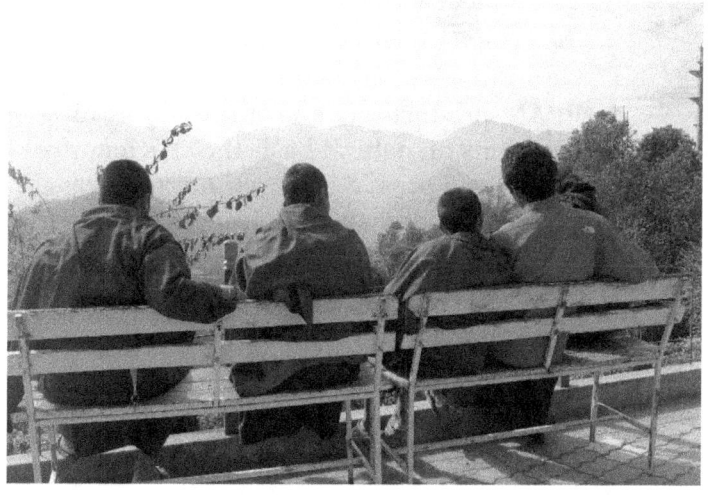

Any information on work of B. Tichanovsky and
efficiency of EPAM herbal preparations
Veronika Malkova
mobile: 00420 606 451 044
www.epam.eu
(English version coming soon...)

EPAM products are one of the few healing
preparations on natural basis the efficiency of
which has been proved by two thousand years of
practice in the past and clinical studies at the
present time.

www.ingramcontent.com/pod-product-compliance
Lightning Source LLC
Chambersburg PA
CBHW070123290526
45789CB00005B/2129

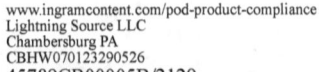